# THE LITTLE BOOK OF
# CRYSTAL
# HEALING

### CATHERINE GERDES

summersdale

THE LITTLE BOOK OF CRYSTAL HEALING

An Hachette UK Company
www.hachette.co.uk

Summersdale Publishers Ltd
Part of Octopus Publishing Group Limited
Carmelite House
50 Victoria Embankment
LONDON
EC4Y 0DZ
UK

www.summersdale.com

Printed and bound in China

ISBN: 978-1-83799-132-7

Substantial discounts on bulk quantities of Summersdale books are available to corporations, professional associations and other organizations. For details contact general enquiries: telephone: +44 (0) 1243 771107 or email: enquiries@summersdale.com.

# CONTENTS

# INTRODUCTION

You may have heard the phrase, "Everything is energy." This is the basis for understanding crystals, including their popularity and purpose. Over millennia, their global significance has been recognized by multiple cultures in healing rituals. However, not every crystal has the same healing themes and, just as they look different and express a wide range of colours, they each hold a variety of meanings.

In this book, we'll explore the wonderful world of crystals and their unique curative properties, so that you can better understand how to integrate them into your own life. Because when combined with intention, crystals are more than just pretty stones – they can become tools for achieving your own unique healing and growth.

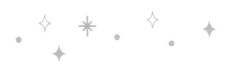

Perhaps you chose this book because you have previously experienced some kind of sensation or change in the presence of crystals. Maybe you've felt soothed by rose quartz, or compelled to hold a shiny, spiky amethyst. You could be negotiating challenging life events and wondering how crystals could help you move through grief or trauma. Or you might never have been in contact with crystals before but are simply curious about things you've heard. However you've found yourself here, welcome to this healing path and the resonating energy of crystals.

This book will guide you in selecting, cleansing and understanding these beautiful stones and their meanings. You'll learn how to work with gems in useful ways, infusing your life with intentionality and, along the journey, discover more about yourself – and the potential of crystals to play a significant role in restoring your energy. These precious gems are more than kaleidoscopic décor. They are earth's special gifts.

*Crystals are
the flowers of the
mineral kingdom.*

EDWARD ABBEY

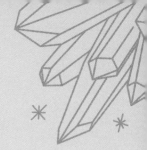

# CHAPTER ONE:

# **THE HISTORY OF CRYSTAL HEALING**

Across millennia, crystals have been historically significant in many cultures. Spanning six continents, both ancient and modern civilizations have accessed their healing properties, using them in rituals performed by Ancient Sumerians and for ornamental wear by the early Egyptians. They were used by the Ancient Greeks and Romans to enhance athletic vitality, and indigenous peoples across North America valued their protective properties. These civilizations collectively understood that specific stones held different potencies and themes and, separately, used them to assist in processing grief, undergoing transformation, cultivating creativity and much more. Let's take a look at some of these practices in more detail.

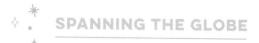

Throughout history, crystals have been used for healing purposes the world over. Here are some of the most notable examples:

## MESOPOTAMIA

Some of the first recorded references to the use of crystals are from the Ancient Sumerians. They are said to have used gemstones in ritualistic practices and medicinal substances, with recordings dating back to between 4500 and 2000 BCE. Like many cultures, the Sumerians made connections between the metaphysical properties of crystals and relief from illness and for personal longevity. They also used stones for protection and to ward off evil within their communities.

## CHINA

In Chinese medicine, the use of crystals is documented in the earliest known records. From 300 BCE, the *Huangdi Neijing* (literally, The Inner Canon of the Yellow Emperor) is an ancient treatise detailing traditional Chinese medicine concepts, which remains the foundation for modern-day practice. Although this system is believed to have existed for thousands of years, the texts outline several important principles for healing and refer to the energies of the natural world, including crystals.

## ANCIENT GREECE

Ancient Greek soldiers and sailors used crystals for protection in battle – the use of hematite, for example, was believed to make one invincible. The Greeks gave names to many of the crystals that we still use today. In fact, the word "crystal" derives from the Greek word for ice, or *krystallos*, as it was believed that crystals were permanently frozen pieces of water. Greek mythology shares the tale of the creation of amethyst, in which an intoxicated Dionysus turns a young girl into clear stone. The story goes that as Dionysus cried into his wine in shame, his cup spilled onto the stone, staining it purple and creating the popular gem.

In 360 BCE, the Greek philosopher, Plato, wrote a work entitled *Timaeus*, in which he described Atlantis, off the north coast of Africa. On this island, crystal healing is mentioned, and he writes about using these gems in intuitive and metaphysical ways. Although presented as fiction, there has been continued fascination surrounding this work's topics and locale in the Eye of the Sahara.

A student of Plato, the Greek philosopher, Theophrastus, wrote one of the first known works devoted to gemstones, titled *Peri Lithon* (Of Stones).

A turquoise given
by a loving hand carries
with it happiness and
good fortune.

**ARABIC PROVERB**

## ANCIENT EGYPT

The Ancient Egyptians are known to have worn crystals – such as lapis lazuli, emerald and carnelian – in their jewellery for protection and health. Evidence of their use of crystals spans from 3100 to 300 BCE. Crystals were incorporated into the sacred passage of ancestors and leaders into the afterlife, and it was believed the mystical energy of crystals would aid in this transition. As an example, in the Egyptian story of Osiris, malachite was used to assist journeys into the underworld, and today this is still a stone associated with transformation. Crystal shapes held significance, too, as stones formed into scarabs were thought to be more protective and used in some burials.

Egyptian royalty, including Cleopatra, used the crushed powder of stones, such as lapis lazuli, for eye make-up, while other stones were crushed to form brightly coloured paint for murals and tombs. Pharaohs and priests utilized quartz to balance specific energy within the body, with hematite used to treat inflammation, while clear quartz was fused into monuments.

## INDIA

Ancient Vedic texts from India refer to the use of crystals for multiple purposes. Although these texts span from 1500 to 1000 BCE, they are still used today in alternative wellness therapies offered worldwide. These texts, referred to as the *Vedas*, are composed of the *Rig-Veda* (for recitation), *Yajur-Veda* (for liturgy), *Sama-Veda* (for chanting) and *Atharva-Veda* (magic formulas).

In these works, as well as biblical ones, ruby is regarded as one of the most precious ancient stones, while diamond, emerald and bloodstone are also referenced in the Vedas. In one specific text, *Garuda Purana – Achara Khanda*, some gemstones are shared for the absolving of sins and for healing from snake bites. In the late nineteenth and early twentieth centuries, modern developments highlight gemstone use further for different forms of relief. Various specific crystals are recommended for balancing Ayurveda's three energy types, called *doshas*, and treating medical ailments. For example, pearl, diamond and moonstone assist with balancing the fiery *pitta dosha*, which can be tied to inflammation when out of balance.

## ANCIENT ROME

Pliny the Elder, the Roman philosopher and author, attributes healing values to each crystal in his encyclopedic text *Natural History*, completed in 77 CE, which classified stones by their colour and appearance. He is considered to be the first to document the similarities between some stones, such as beryl and emerald. However, although a notable historical work, it is believed that some of these gemstone descriptions were actually passed down and not from his personal experience.

Both before and after the Common Era – specifically between 27 BCE and 476 CE – the Romans used crystals as amulets and talismans to provide protection in battle, and attract health and good fortune into their personal lives. Crystals were also used in Roman medical treatments, such as supporting safe childbirth and easing indigestion.

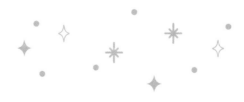

## CYPRUS

In 350 CE, Saint Epiphanius, Bishop of Salamis in Cyprus, wrote about the twelve stones in the breastplate of the high priest from the Bible's book of Exodus. This was the first biblical mention of a lapidary – the referencing of stones in a text – and those cited include carnelian, chrysolite, beryl, turquoise, lapis lazuli, emerald, jacinth, agate, amethyst, topaz, onyx and jasper. The bishop assigns therapeutic virtues to each stone. Additionally, the Bible references rubies in the New Testament, sapphires in the Old Testament, and clear crystals in both. Despite this, biblical texts do not assign metaphysical properties to gemstones. However, throughout the Middle Ages, Christians ascribed bloodstone (so called due to its resemblance to droplets of Jesus's blood during the crucifixion) with sacred healing abilities.

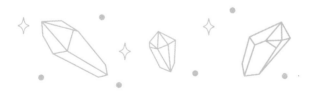

## SPAIN

Saint Isidore, the archbishop of Seville, wrote *Etymologiarum sive Originum libri XX,* an encyclopedic work that famously shared gemstone data and descriptions, which became a reference material for subsequent centuries. Throughout the Middle Ages, this text influenced public knowledge surrounding crystals, as well as their general acceptance for metaphysical use.

In 1253, Alfonso X, the Spanish king famous for his writings and musical compositions, wrote about the connections between gemstones and astrology in a manuscript called *Lapidary of Alfonso X the Wise.* In this work, he shares metaphysical and medical healing information related to gemstones and includes astrological depictions.

## FRANCE

Marbod, the Bishop of Rennes from the eleventh century, is known for his influential *Liber de Lapidibus.* Comprising more than a hundred poetic manuscripts, it references the earliest lapidary of the Middle Ages. The work delves into the formation of stones, as well as highlighting more healing properties, such as beryl for the liver and agate for the eyes.

## GERMANY

In 1260, German philosopher Saint Albert the Great, or Albertus Magnus, wrote the treatise *De Mineralibus* (On Minerals). In this notable work, he offered a scientific perspective on the use of crystals in healing practices. Structured in five sections, with some devoted to stones and others to metals, it was informed by his first-hand experience and extensive travel, as he encountered many minerals and miners during the thousands of miles traversed.

## WIDER EUROPE

Throughout the Renaissance in Europe, precious and semi-precious stones were used in herbal remedies to treat the sick. Apothecaries would display decorative crystals in curiosity cabinets in geometric patterns. In addition to superficially displayed gems, they would utilize minerals to create medicines. Likewise, royal court physicians made concoctions that incorporated minerals for healing. This growing interest in gemstones correlated with the invention of the printing press. Several alchemical works were published, enabling the information to reach wider audiences, which subsequently fostered a renewed interest in the healing properties of crystals.

## THE AMERICAS

From the past to the present day, indigenous peoples of the Americas have revered the natural world, using crystals for a variety of purposes, including the wearing of turquoise for strength and spiritual connection, or keeping a black onyx talisman for protection. Different types of quartz were used by some indigenous tribes for various reasons. For example, rose quartz was known for its curative properties, while clear quartz was carried or worn for positive luck. The Hopi of modern-day Arizona use quartz for healing and diagnosing illnesses, while Mayans and Aztecs collected and utilized obsidian, which was plentiful, for protection and Shamanic rituals. In addition to ornamental or medicinal uses, some stones were favoured for tools and weaponry.

Most indigenous traditions are orally taught and kept close within the community but, as with their honouring of nature itself, their respect for, and use of, crystals is well known.

## JAPAN

People of Japan have also connected with crystals, turning to them for their intuitive properties and ability to offer clarity. Historically, they have been linked to clairvoyance and also used to *scry* (the practice of reading crystals for prophetic purposes). Clear quartz is particularly valued and has been tied to Japanese mythology. Symbolizing dragon's breath, it is associated with generosity, wisdom and perfection. But jadeite, or *hisui*, may be the most prized stone, both in antiquity and today, as it was selected as the national stone of Japan in 2016 and has been unearthed from ancient burial tombs. One of the world's largest jadeite boulders is a modern-day UNESCO heritage site in Itoigawa.

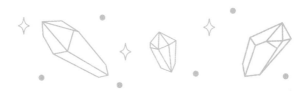

# CRYSTAL SCEPTICISM

During the Age of Enlightenment, Thomas Nicols published *Gemmarius Fidelius* (The Faithful Lapidary). In this work from the 1650s, Nicols denied the metaphysical characteristics and healing abilities of gemstones. His perspective contributed to the diminished public interest in crystals across parts of Europe.

As scepticism grew around crystal healing in the mid-1800s, investigations increased into crystal and faith healers. This, coupled with scientific advances, led people towards new medicinal quests and steered them away from curiosity around gemstones. Despite this widespread suspicion, in 1880, the French physicists Jacques and Pierre Curie, known as the Curie brothers, recorded an electric charge that was evident from quartz, which came to be known as the *piezoelectric effect*. In 1921, Walter Guyton Cady patented the first quartz crystal oscillator, which became widely used in radios and other technologic devices. It is still in use today.

# THE FUTURE OF CRYSTALS

Despite this notable and global timeline, we've only scratched the surface of the chronology of healing crystals! As you can see, they have a rich historical track record. In fact, having formed over millions of years, they *are* history itself.

While crystals are interwoven into many cultures, with this affinity passed down through generations, the fascination with crystals has been revitalized for modern-day spiritual well-being. Today, we're seeing a renaissance that mirrors the fascination of the 1960s and 1970s, when there was a popular fascination with mind, body, spirit healing and the mystical properties of crystals, alongside astrology. This has been referred to as the advent of New Age culture. While the decades that followed were a quieter period of reduced interest in crystal healing, we are currently witnessing a growing resurgence of alternative medicine and therapies, including forms of energy healing work.

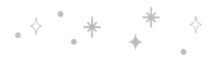

*Colour is a power
which directly
influences the soul.*

**WASSILY KANDINSKY**

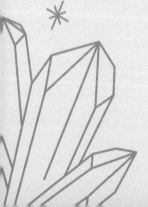

# A HISTORY OF COLOUR

Using colour in wellness practices has early Egyptian and Chinese origins, as it was understood to improve well-being. In Ancient Egypt, colour was used to treat illness, with some hues associated with deities and themes, such as black symbolizing fertility and gold representing eternity. Colour is also used in Chinese medicine, linked to various organ systems. For example, green is tied to the liver, while yellow is connected to the spleen.

Colour therapy, or chromotherapy, incorporates colour and light to produce emotional, mental and physical benefits. In *The Spectro-Chrome Metry Encyclopedia*, written in 1933 by Dinshah P. Ghadiali, the author explains how colour has the capability to bring healing to imbalances in the body and elevate mood, and these findings are still used today.

Some of the emotional colour correspondences from colour therapy are detailed below. Outside of this specific treatment, there are many ways to incorporate the use of colour into your daily life, such as surrounding yourself with the colour that correlates to the emotional experience you're seeking. Of course, another powerful way to access these benefits is working with crystals of appropriate hues.

- **Red** is stimulating and has the ability to energize or provoke nervousness.

- **Orange** can evoke joy, move energy, and is associated with appetite and creativity.

- **Yellow** is connected to happiness and can provide a boost of positivity.

- **Green** is associated with the natural world and has soothing effects.

- **Blue** is used for relaxation and can be stress reducing, but it specifically targets pain and sadness.

- **Purple** is tied to spiritual awareness and is used for connecting with higher knowledge and dissolving mental stress.

# PREVALENT CRYSTALS IN HISTORY

We've had an overview of the various ways crystals have been used throughout history. Now, let's look more closely at some stones with fascinating histories from around the world...

## JADE

Highly regarded in Ancient Chinese culture, jade has been carved into musical chimes and used for the burial rituals of Chinese emperors. Some Chinese written characters were influenced by jade, and it has also been associated with healing of the kidneys in both Chinese and Mayan culture. In New Zealand, jade is similarly revered and believed to hold strong ties to one's ancestry. In Mayan and Japanese society, a rare form of this stone is referred to as *jadeite* and celebrated and used in a variety of ways. And while the Mayans also used it in burials, this practice was adopted from their ancestral culture, the Olmec. The Mayans used jadeite for décor and adornment, in sculpture, jewellery and tooth inlays.

## ROSE QUARTZ

Rose quartz was revered in Ancient Egypt for its ability to slow the ageing process and was used for superficial beautification, while Ancient Romans used it for embossed seals on documents, to finalize agreements. Today, rose quartz is widely valued as a stone representing love, and is often used to mend heartbreak, harmonize emotions and heal relationships.

## CARNELIAN

This stone's name is derived from the Latin word *Carneus*, meaning fleshy, and refers to the quality of its hue. It was treasured and fashioned into amulets in Ancient Egypt and used by the Ancient Sumerians in decorative jewellery, signet rings and seals. The Ancient Romans and Greeks also utilized carnelian for rings as a symbol of status and, as with a few other specific stones, it was considered to offer safe passage for ancestors into the afterlife.

## BLACK GEMSTONES

Various black gemstones carry tales of protective intrigue and personal adornment. Nuummite, a black metallic speckled stone native to Greenland, is one of the oldest known minerals in the world and thought to be a strong, energetic protector.

Known for its sharpness, obsidian was used in arrowheads by many indigenous peoples, as well as in traditional Aztec wooden clubs, called *Macuahuitl*.

In Pliny the Elder's work, he shared the curative properties of jet, which included healing toothache and targeting tumours. Jet was also used during the Stone Age for its metaphysical protective qualities.

Onyx was noted as one of the stones prized for authenticating seals in Ancient Mesopotamia, and was popular in forming cameos – carved accessories worn within the Roman Empire. They were also commissioned and gifted to others by Napoleon, depicting his profile with an onyx backdrop.

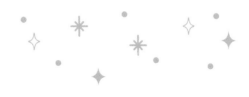

## AGATE

Given its name by the Greek philosopher, Theophrastus, this stone was first documented along the Sicilian shoreline but can be found worldwide. In fact, it was reported in the German Nahe region during the reign of Julius Caesar, with the largest quantities in southern Brazil. One of its more costly forms is dendritic agate. This stone aesthetically mimics plants and was linked to Artemis, the Greek goddess of the hunt, who is closely associated with forests.

## MALACHITE

From Russian palace columns to striking American vases, rich, green-banded malachite has found its way into larger-than-life and lavish settings the world over. Admired for its pigment, it was used in paints during the Renaissance era. In Ancient Egypt, malachite symbolized fertility and new life, and was used in make-up by Egyptian royalty. During Medieval times, its protective powers were harnessed by doting parents, who placed it on their children's beds to ward off evil.

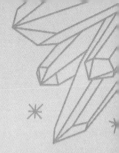

# CHAPTER TWO:

## CRYSTAL HEALING 101

Crystals are a tool to help us restore our energy. But in order to understand healing with crystals, you must also understand your body and the flow of energy within it. Just as we went back through the ages to learn about crystal formation and use, we must return to ancient practices to study the process of working with crystals.

By the end of this chapter, you'll become familiar with this system, and know how to select, cleanse, charge and care for your new crystal collection. But before delving further into our relationship with gemstones, we'll start by better understanding ourselves.

# CRYSTALS AND THE CHAKRAS

Remember our *Everything is energy* saying? This includes ourselves and is reflected through a system called the *chakras*. Originating in Ancient India, this system was documented in ancient Vedic texts, which are the basis for Hinduism today. But they have influenced many outside this one religion, and energy centres have been recognized by various cultures, including the indigenous peoples of the Americas, as well as the Chinese, Sufis and Egyptians.

The word *chakra* comes from the Sanskrit word, *chakram* (wheel), because these centres are meant to be spinning like a wheel to move energy through the body. This energetic system is aligned with the spine and moves beyond it. Just as our physical bodies are alike, the chakras are similarly found in person to person, each holding different meanings with a range of associations, including crystals. As you learn about each chakra, it can guide your decision-making process when selecting crystals.

## THE ROOT CHAKRA

**Sanskrit name:** *Muladhara*
**Colour:** Red
**Location:** Base of the spine

The first chakra is the root chakra, which is tied to themes of stability, independence and feelings of security. Crystals for this chakra are intended to support our feelings of safety and presence in the here and now. The root chakra is connected to our survival instincts. You may notice that the stones for the root chakra are all deep hues and mostly rich, earthy tones. These shades are reminiscent of the earth beneath our feet. Protective and grounding, the black stones are also associated with this chakra. Some of the crystals for healing this chakra include bloodstone, red jasper, black tourmaline and shungite. For crystal meditations, these stones can be placed on the bladder, thighs, surrounding you while seated, or placed on the floor beneath your feet. You can also carry one of these stones on you throughout the day, such as in your pocket. However, you don't have to keep it near the chakra to receive its healing properties.

**Root chakra affirmation:** I am safe and secure being me.

## THE SACRAL CHAKRA

**Sanskrit name:** *Svadhisthana*
**Colour:** Orange
**Location:** Below the navel

Following the grounding work of the root chakra, we have the second, or sacral, chakra. This chakra is connected to our sensuality and creativity. Sacral energy can be tied to satisfying our creative genius or the whims of our inner child. Crystals for this chakra are intended to support our connection with pleasure, expression and natural enthusiasm. Sacral chakra stones can also help maintain good or high energy levels – just thinking of their vibrant orange or rich brown tones can evoke an energetic boost! Some of the crystals for the sacral chakra include carnelian, tiger's eye, moonstone, fire agate and orange calcite. When meditating with these stones, you'll want to place them around the lower abdomen or over the bladder. Working on the neighbouring root chakra can also impact your sacral energy.

**Sacral chakra affirmation:** I am free to express myself creatively. I celebrate my uniqueness.

## THE SOLAR PLEXUS

**Sanskrit name:** *Manipura*
**Colour:** Yellow
**Location:** Above the navel

Our third chakra is the solar plexus (physically, a collection of nerves in the abdomen), which is connected to our self-esteem and ego. Crystals for this chakra are great for helping us to tackle insecurity and encourage joy or, conversely, they can help us address excessive pride. Working with solar plexus energies can help us express ourselves more authentically. If you're seeking to summon the courage for public speaking or a big announcement, solar plexus crystals might be a good choice. Some of these include agate, citrine, yellow jasper, yellow topaz and pyrite. When meditating on solar plexus healing with crystals, you will want to place these on the upper portion of the abdomen and just below the chest. You might also position them prominently in your living area or workspace.

**Solar plexus chakra affirmation:** I stand in alignment with my truest self and find inner strength.

Nothing can
dim the light that
shines from within.

**MAYA ANGELOU**

## THE HEART CHAKRA

**Sanskrit name:** *Anahata*
**Colour:** Green
**Location:** Centre of the chest

The heart chakra is a key chakra to concentrate on, given that it focuses on healing emotions of the past and present, and helps us cultivate healthy relationships. As its name suggests, crystals for the heart chakra are intended to support reciprocal love and the self-healing of past traumas or grief. It doesn't only cover interpersonal relationships but also includes our relationship with ourselves. Heart-related crystals are some of the most popular, and there are many for this chakra, but the most well-recognized include rose quartz, aventurine, malachite, moss agate and jade. For meditations with the heart, hold or place your crystal over the centre of your chest. You could also wear a heart-healing crystal on a pendant over this chakra.

**Heart chakra affirmation:** I am worthy of love, joy and inner peace.

## THE THROAT CHAKRA

**Sanskrit name:** *Vishuddha*
**Colour:** Turquoise
**Location:** Centre of the throat

The fifth chakra is the throat chakra, which contains themes of communication and expression of the truth. Crystals for this chakra are intended to support practices such as speaking up for yourself and not suppressing your voice. They are also connected to our capacity to hold space, by listening attentively to others. Some of the crystals for the throat chakra that are supportive of our expression of truth include aquamarine, celestite, turquoise, blue lace agate and blue topaz. To work with this chakra in meditation, place any of these stones over or around the throat and allow its soothing energies to free up the space for your truth to come forth. You might also consider a choker necklace with your throat-related stone for support.

**Throat chakra affirmation:** I express my truth freely, with honesty and integrity.

## THE THIRD EYE CHAKRA

**Sanskrit name:** *Ajna*
**Colour:** Indigo
**Location:** Between the eyebrows

Our third eye chakra is the sixth chakra. The themes for this centre are intuition and inner knowing. When working with the third eye, crystals are meant to help develop intuition and trust. These are meant to support us in our natural understanding, without having concrete proof. Some crystals that support this chakra include lapis lazuli, labradorite, moldavite, tanzanite and unakite. For meditations with the third eye, gently place your chosen crystal between your brows on your forehead. Like the heart chakra, the third eye is sensitive. You might want to start with a smaller stone or one that feels more "subtle" to you. Or you may choose to place a third eye crystal under your pillow while you sleep.

**Third eye affirmation:** I trust my vision and am open to receiving guidance from the universe.

## THE CROWN CHAKRA

**Sanskrit name:** *Sahasrara*
**Colour:** Purple
**Location:** Top of the head

Finally, our seventh chakra is tied to themes of spirituality, divinity and collective consciousness. The crown is the opposite of the grounding root chakra, as it connects us to the universal consciousness that transcends the self. Similar to the third eye, crystal use for the crown is intended for connection to our intuition and the divine, utilizing crystals that include selenite, clear quartz, opal, lepidolite and beryl. To work with the crown chakra, first place grounding stones around the feet, root chakra or around your seat. Then, position the crown chakra crystal of your choice just above or on the head. You can also sleep with crown chakra crystals beneath your pillow, for support and connection.

**Crown chakra affirmation:** I move forward in openness and trust. I am ready to receive.

## CRYSTALS AND THE PHYSICAL BODY

Ancient practitioners believed the energy of certain crystals corresponded to the healing of particular organ systems within the body. The subtle energies of these specific crystals are believed to encourage the healing process of these structures:

✦ **Brain and memory:** citrine, yellow fluorite, green calcite, azurite

✦ **Eyes:** blue lace agate, jade, malachite, lapis lazuli

✦ **Throat, ears and thyroid:** beryl, aquamarine, lapis lazuli, amazonite

✦ **Heart:** rose quartz, kunzite, rhodonite

✦ **Gallbladder:** yellow jasper, amber, carnelian

✦ **Liver:** hematite, bloodstone, tiger's eye

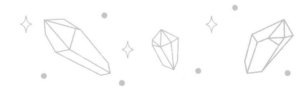

- **Gut health:** amethyst, citrine, carnelian
- **Reproductive organs:** jasper, carnelian, tiger's eye
- **Immune system:** green tourmaline, clear quartz, selenite
- **Skin:** aquamarine, rose quartz, jade

In addition, specific stones that target the reduction of inflammation include moss agate, larimar, rhodonite, lapis lazuli and clear quartz. Please note that crystals aren't intended to replace the healing work of a medical professional.

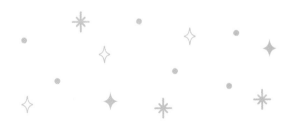

# THE ORIGIN OF CRYSTALS

Crystals are beautiful – but how do they arrive in our hands? Let's go back to basics, to discover a crystal's origin story.

Crystals are created in various ways the world over, and can take millions of years to form – some layer by layer, through the gradual accumulation of matter under pressure, while others form as a result of subterranean drainage and drips, which eventually crystalize. In a nutshell, when molecules gradually amass into a solid structure because of the process of liquid hardening, the earth forms a crystal.

Crystals have various structures which are formed in diverse temperatures and environments but all are organic compounds that require time to evolve. Some are abundant while others are scarce and, in some cases, requiring tremendous effort to source.

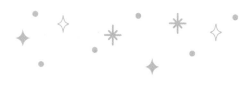

## PRECIOUS VERSUS SEMI-PRECIOUS STONES

What makes one crystal easy to purchase, while others, like diamonds, are a significant investment? Crystals can be divided into two categories, recognized since the mid-nineteenth century – precious and semi-precious. The difference is determined by physical attributes, reputation and rarity, which impacts cost.

There are just four precious stones – diamond, ruby, sapphire and emerald. Precious stones are typically transparent and faceted. Despite a price difference, semi-precious stones are not inferior to precious stones and include most of the essential crystals we'll cover, with examples including moonstone, agate, carnelian and amethyst.

## MINERALS

A mineral is a naturally occurring crystalline structure that has not been cut or polished. Most gemstones are derived from minerals. There are fake gemstones created in laboratories, but while these can be gems, they are not minerals, because they did not come from the earth and are not organic compounds. Examples of these synthetic gems are cubic zirconia or imitation emerald.

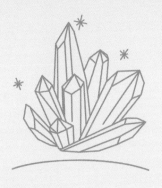

FORMED OVER
MILLIONS OF YEARS,
CRYSTALS ARE
PIECES OF HISTORY
IN YOUR HANDS

## ETHICAL SOURCING

Considering the history of crystal mining and working conditions, it's important to make ethical sourcing a part of your selection process. Since these stones are sourced the world over and some locales have inhumane working conditions, it's vital to bring conscious awareness to how your crystals reach you – and how they are being acquired. Some purveyors of precious stones share this information on their websites. Always make sure you purchase crystals from a reputable seller. When in doubt, you can always ask about issues surrounding the safety of working conditions, the involvement of child labour and environmental impact. With the escalating popularity of stones, this continues to be an important topic.

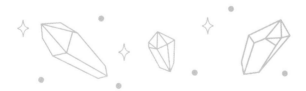

# CRYSTALS BY TYPE

Crystals come in a variety of shapes. Some appear perfectly cut, while others maintain raw, rough edges. Maybe you have felt drawn to one type or form over another. Various shapes hold different properties, which can inform their use.

+ **Cluster** – clusters can be small or large, but they are often raw, meaning they aren't cut or faceted. These are great for holding in meditation, using as a meaningful trinket or placed around the home.

+ **Point** – points are often used for crystal grids (see page 68), on or around the body during meditation or as decorative accents. These have a defined point which is faceted, while the other end is usually rougher and more uncut. The pointed end directs the energy and, in a grid, this can be used to aim it with intention, such as towards yourself or out into your home.

◆ **Pyramid** – similar to crystal points, the apex of a pyramid concentrates and directs energy, but it has a flat base. Crystal pyramids are useful for setting intentions and for display.

◆ **Slab** – crystal slabs are used to decorate a space and subtly influence its energy. These can be utilized as "charging stations" for other crystals, heightening their healing properties. Agate often comes in slabs.

◆ **Geode** – these usually look like smooth rocks that have been broken open to reveal rough interior edges. They sometimes resemble fantastical dinosaur eggs or mystical caves, and are mostly seen with amethyst. Geodes are frequently used for influencing the energy of a space.

◆ **Ball** – this is a spherical crystal which comes in a variety of sizes. Historically used for scrying or forecasting, the ball emits energy equally in all directions and can be placed on pedestals or simply held in your hand.

◆ **Square** – these crystal cubes are ideal for keeping in a space to influence the grounding nature within it. Square shapes are most often seen with pyrite and root chakra stones.

◆ **Egg** – as the name suggests, crystal eggs are cylindrical and perfect for holding in your hand while sitting in meditation. The shape tends to have a soothing effect. A variety of different types of crystals can be turned into an egg shape.

◆ **Wands** – these have been traditionally used by shamans, and can be faceted (artificially shaped) or naturally formed. Crystal wands are great for keeping in a space for energy healing work, and are commonly utilized with a clear intention. Whether for personal or professional use, wands can swipe and clear the aura around and above the body.

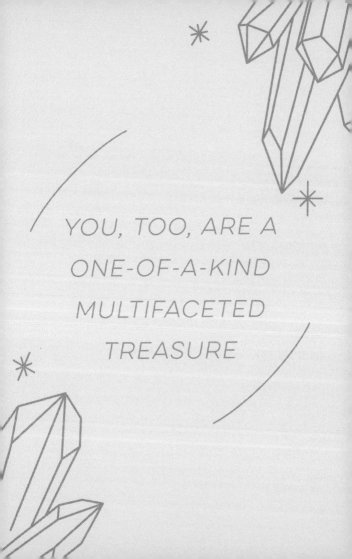

YOU, TOO, ARE A
ONE-OF-A-KIND
MULTIFACETED
TREASURE

# HOW TO SELECT YOUR CRYSTALS

There are a few different approaches for selecting your crystals. The first method is how many people initiate their gem-loving journey — by relying on intuition. After all, this process should be fun, not a burden!

## SELECTING BY INTUITION

We all emit vibrational energy, so you might feel drawn towards one specific crystal. For example, if you're grieving the loss of a loved one, you may be magnetically attracted towards a piece of rhodonite. Or if you're in a depressive funk and in need of a lift, some citrine point or sunstone jewellery could provide the right fit. When you select crystals using your intuition, it's the perfect opportunity to look up the meaning of that crystal. This practice is also a method for developing self-trust.

## SELECTING BY HEALING PROPERTY

Another way to select your crystals is through their healing attributes. This starts with an acknowledgement of any emotional or physical symptoms you're experiencing, before finding crystals with the properties that are aligned with your specific ailments. This is a prescriptive method of selecting stones.

## SELECTING BY CHAKRA THEMES

Now you're familiar with the chakras and their different themes, you may choose to select crystals based on which chakra (or physical part of you) needs the most love and attention. This can be the best route if you're feeling drawn towards multiple crystals of a specific colour, instead of a single stone. If a specific part of your body is in need of restoration, this can also be a good tactic.

In addition to these methods, your choices can be determined by other factors, such as cost, availability or personal preference.

# A CRYSTAL'S NATURE

Before being sourced and made available for your personal collection, it's important to note that crystals might be static, but their energy is not. As part of the natural world, they are constantly drawing energy from it. Whether in the form of cleansing storms, radiant sunlight or in the process of being formed beneath the earth's strata, they are naturally clearing, charging and being cultivated – but they don't remain static.

Crystals are meant to be *incorporated* into your world. This means they are not meant to remain stored away inside a box or ignored on a dusty shelf. This disregard literally neglects the energy and keeps it stuck or dull, instead of vibrant, impactful and flowing. If you've had trouble connecting with crystals, this could be because neglect of the stones left them lacklustre. They need to be nurtured. Fortunately, this doesn't require too much effort.

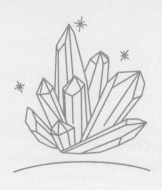

# CRYSTALS ARE
# EARTH'S NATURAL
# MASTERPIECES

# CARING FOR CRYSTALS

Since your new crystals are carrying energy, it's a good idea to cleanse them before you begin working with them. In their journey to you, they will have been in contact with different people from the past – so this energy needs to be refreshed and cleared. There are a variety of ways to do it, but whichever method you choose, setting your intention to clear the energy is an important part of the process.

One common method for resetting the energy of crystals is through the use of cleansing herbs. Not everyone selling these will be ethically sourcing them or practising eco-friendly harvesting, so you'll need to ask whichever vendor you're working with. Pass your crystals through the smoke of the lit herbs of your choice to cleanse old energy.

In some instances, water can be used for this purpose – simply leave the stone immersed in a bowl or pass it through running water. But don't assume every stone can be cleansed this way. When in doubt, research that particular stone or ask the vendor.

Some crystals don't need clearing, although we would still recommend cleansing when you initially acquire them. These crystals are known to be self-clearing, and can even clear the energy of other crystals – such as clear quartz, selenite, carnelian, citrine and kyanite.

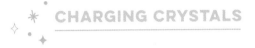

## CHARGING CRYSTALS

Once you've cleared your crystals, you'll want to charge them. This is a way of hyping up their energy, or supporting their natural essence. Charging can be done before and between the times you're working with them. If you wear your crystals, you'll want to do this periodically. The schedule should really be determined by you, but if they're emitting dull vibes, it can be an indicator they need a little loving care.

Charging can be done through natural elements. Using sunlight gives a natural boost to their energy. Clear quartz, or clear stones, are perfect for charging in the sun. You can do this for a brief duration, such as a few minutes outside, or leave them on a windowsill for several hours during the day. Either way, you might instinctively sense the appropriate amount of time for your crystals. However, some crystals are visibly impacted by sunlight and their colour will fade from this exposure. You'll want to check this before resorting to the sun as the energy boost for your gems.

If you can't charge them in sunlight, moonlight is also commonly used instead.

## THE MOON AND CRYSTALS

In the Essential Crystals guide (from page 93), you'll find suggested practices, some of which involve the two main moon phases – the new moon and the full moon. In your personalized practices, you can work with crystals in sync with these moon cycles, utilizing specific crystals. When incorporating crystals in any ritual, you'll want to cleanse and charge them in advance. Or you may choose to use these powerful windows to do so. To charge your crystals during either the new or full moon, cleanse them first, then lay them out on a mat or towel in the moonlight, on a windowsill or outside. You may even decide to leave these in a potted plant, or in the soil.

## THE NEW MOON

This is a good time for setting intentions and gaining clarity. New moons can be an opportunity to explore what really matters – and to ask ourselves if we're acting in alignment with what we truly desire. Just as the moon is hidden from sight during this phase, we may have to search for what we've kept concealed. This energy evokes a combination of working with the subconscious and strategizing how to take action.

## THE FULL MOON

When all of the moon is clearly visible and the sky is brightest at night it is called a full moon. Just as the light of the moon illuminates, it's an ideal time to see what is being revealed. Between the new and full moons, the moon's strength and brightness are building, providing opportunities for harnessing this energy for manifestations – particularly around releasing. It's often a period of letting something go. This can be personal, such as a habit or thought pattern. Full moons can be highly charged windows of time to release stuck emotions and allow ourselves to feel, so try to avoid distractions or suppression of your feelings.

Often affiliated with feminine energy, there are specific stones tied to the sensitive, cyclical energy of the moon. Some of these include moonstone, celestite, angelite, selenite and labradorite.

## PUTTING IT TOGETHER

Now you understand the energies associated with these two main moon cycles, you can begin working with them. Start by cleansing your stones in the way that feels most appropriate for you and is best for maintaining them. Then, you might consider laying them out on a soft surface overnight during a full moon. Resting a towel beneath them or placing them outside over grass or in dirt is also effective. Some prefer to nestle their stones in soil or bury them – you might try this for 12 to 24 hours. If you've chosen to charge your crystals during a full moon, you'll want to simply make sure the gems are able to bask in its light. You'll likely notice the difference in your gemstones the following day. This recharge can allow you to work with them again, through wearing them, meditating with them or strategically placing them within your home.

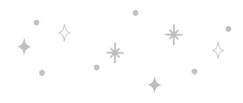

The goal of life is
living in agreement
with nature.

**ZENO**

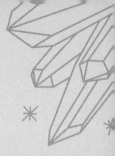

CHAPTER THREE:

# HOW TO USE CRYSTALS FOR HEALING

You don't need the fanciest precious stone jewellery or an impressive standing amethyst in your home to sense and receive the benefits of gemstones. As you'll have learned in the previous chapters, stones have historically been carried in the form of protective pieces, which provides an easy route to begin working with them. Instead of feeling a pressure to incorporate crystals in some regimented way into your life, you could simply begin keeping them in your pocket and noticing the sensations they provide. Or you could create personalized rituals that feel right for you. The following pages will help you get this process started.

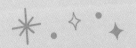

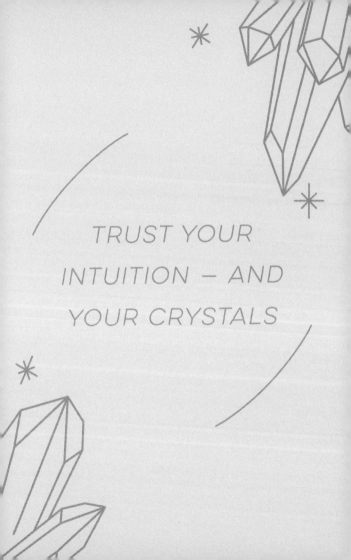

TRUST YOUR
INTUITION — AND
YOUR CRYSTALS

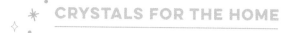

# CRYSTALS FOR THE HOME

The incorporation of specific crystals can help your space feel light, serene and secure. But before placing crystals around your home, you'll want to clear the space first.

Literally cleaning and decluttering the area is a good place to start. Then, use the smoke of cleansing herbs, allowing natural air to flow through and assist with clearing the energy in your rooms. In addition to crystals and herbs, the natural elements of sunlight and fresh air are also cleansing for the home.

Once this process is complete, you'll want to choose protective and grounding stones. Set the intention for your home to be a place of peace and sanctuary. To maintain good energy, keep clutter to a minimum. This will also help energy flow through your home. In addition to the stones you've used for grounding, keep cleansing and uplifting stones in places that feel right for you.

## WHICH CRYSTALS GO WHERE?

✦ Selenite, black tourmaline or other protective black stones are excellent to keep in various parts of your home. Set up some of these stones around the outer corners of your house and near doorways.

✦ Rose quartz is great for keeping in your bedroom and in spaces where you get ready, dressed or accessorize. Moonstone, jade and amethyst are also supportive of beautification, adornment and inner strength.

✦ Clear quartz is a popular stone for balancing the energy of a space, while amethyst and citrine uplift this energy.

✦ Keeping energizing stones in places where you work or work out can be beneficial. The best crystals for this intention are those connected to the sacral or solar plexus chakras. These stones can include garnet, carnelian or yellow topaz.

## THE SIMPLICITY
## OF TUMBLE STONES

Tumble stones (small, round, highly-polished stones) are a simple way to work with crystals on a daily basis. You can wear them, carry them as a talisman (a signature item which, when coupled with the wearer's intention, offers a sense of energetic security), or place them in significant places around your home. Another way to work with tumble stones is to leave them in places that are important to you. For some, this might be in the car. For others, it could be within workspaces. You might prefer placing them on paperwork, with an intention tied to it. Or you might like leaving oracle or tarot cards out and placing a single gem on top. Whichever way feels natural to use tumble stones – or any crystal – is entirely up to you.

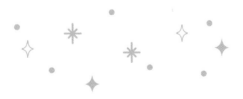

Though we cannot
understand the life of a
crystal, it is nonetheless
a living being.

**NIKOLA TESLA**

# PERFORMING A
# CRYSTAL MEDITATION

Historically, crystals have been used in prayer and meditation. Since their use throughout centuries for medicinal purposes, as recorded in the Vedas and Chinese medical texts, it's not unexpected that we'd use them in meditation, too.

You could try keeping stones with you during your next meditation practice, or you might like to attempt aligning crystals with the chakras in meditation. This is one way to work with crystals alongside your physical body. When you were reading through the chakras, it's likely that at least one of these points and its themes stood out to you to focus on. Using this information, find the crystal that speaks to you, lie down comfortably and rest the corresponding crystal over the chakra you wish to balance.

# TOP TIPS FOR
# CRYSTAL MEDITATION

As energy flows through the chakras from the earth's crystals, it's no surprise that laying stones over specific parts of the body can be a conduit for healing.

To relax into this meditation, focus on your breathing and, without concentrating on any particular thing, notice your thoughts. Any attempts to fix or solve external issues in life should be put to rest for the duration of this exercise. If you choose to focus on any specific topic, allow it to be on the healing of this specific part of your body and the themes that accompany it. Also, give yourself an appropriate amount of time and space alone to perform this. Since you'll be allowing yourself to relax, you may benefit from setting a timer.

# ADDITIONAL MEDITATIONS TO CONSIDER

## CREATE A SOUND BATH WITH OR WITHOUT CRYSTALS

In addition to your meditation, you can set up a sound bath for yourself. This is an experience that utilizes sound waves, for example, in the form of music or tones, for the purposes of healing. If you have trouble unwinding or relaxing, this can be a special salve to help you ease into a meditative practice. Use gentle music or nature sounds and allow them to emit healing vibrations. If you want a different aural experience, you can find an in-person sound healing event and grab a few crystals to bring with you. Or, if you feel intrigued by crystal bowls, you may wish to experiment with one (or some) to accompany your meditations.

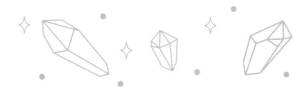

## PERFORM VISUALIZATION WORK

You may want to combine some of your intention-setting work with your crystal healing meditation. In this meditative state, with your eyes closed and the particular crystals of your choosing, paint a mental visualization of a landscape. You might create a dream scenario for yourself. Really see yourself there. Or you might simply start with a mental picture of a particular place and, as you sit with that visual, notice the thoughts it evokes. Which sensations arise? Let your imagination run wild and embrace what unfolds.

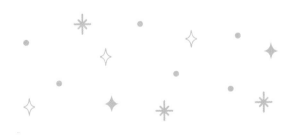

# CRYSTAL GRIDS

Crystal grids involve the deliberate placement of crystals in a space, or around the home or body. Typically, these are beautiful geometric patterns filled with multi-coloured crystals. Grids are used to ground the energy of your intentions, and around the home, or in a physical space, for protection, positivity or inspiration. When positioned around the body while laying down, grids are utilized for healing purposes.

Technically, there are no rules for creating grids. However, the crystals you choose to work with will determine the combined energy. For example, quartz will amplify the energies of other stones, or if one stone is tied to crown chakra themes, a grounding stone will counteract that. Depending on your intentions, this can either be positive, or not serve your intention well.

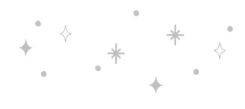

When lying down, grids can be formed by placing crystals around and on the physical body. If you're creating a grid for the body, it is beneficial to use a grounding stone around the ankles or feet. Often, spiritual stones, such as amethyst or quartz, are positioned over the head. Incorporating a grounding stone balances out the vibrational weight, helping you feel more rooted.

Once you've incorporated these two by the feet and above the head, an easy way to create a crystal grid around the body is to follow the chakras. Either place crystals on or surrounding the body that correspond with each of the chakras. Now relax and allow the energy to naturally unfold. Of course, you'll want to cleanse your stones and set intentions ahead of time.

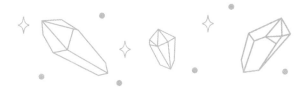

# CREATING YOUR CRYSTAL GRID

To create a crystal grid, begin with a clear intention. For example, you might consider heightening creativity, boosting loving energy, healing the past, or creating peaceful sleep cycles.

Collect eight quartz crystal points and either four or eight other stones of your choosing. You can work with more if you wish, but this is a good place to begin. In addition, select one main stone that signifies the overarching purpose of creating your grid. Aesthetically, you may want this to be your largest stone. As an example, amethyst might work well for this. Start the formation of your grid by placing it in the centre. Using the cardinal directions (north, south, east and west), place your four or eight collected stones in a pattern radiating outwards from the centre stone. When doing this, you may want to take the cardinal directions into consideration, as they contain energetic meanings as well:

✦ North is associated with wisdom

✦ South is tied to action

✦ East is tied to the future

✦ West is connected to reflection and letting go

You may choose to work with these themes in your creation, or to reflect on what they might signify in relation to your intention.

When you've placed the stones that feel right for you in a pattern that radiates out from the central point, finish with your quartz crystal points as the final touch on the "rays" of your crystal grid. The quartz will serve to amplify the energy of the other stones and, placed on the outermost tips of your grid, will radiate it outwards.

Lastly, light a candle or incorporate a natural scent that resonates for you, such as cedarwood, which can feel grounding, or lemon, which is uplifting. Meditate or reflect on your original intention, allowing your crystal grid to gently support your process and remind you of your initial desire.

If you want to simplify this process, start with just one stone centred around your intention and eight quartz points radiating out from this stone, forming a sun-like shape.

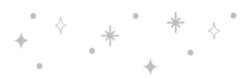

# CRYSTALS AND MOOD

By now, we know crystals, along with other natural elements, work with the mind, body, and spirit in their healing capabilities.

As well as there being specific crystals to heal the physical body, there are also crystals associated with a variety of emotional states, including improving mood. The vibrations from certain stones positively impact our overall well-being. Their healing vibrations affect the subtle body – or the unseen, sensitive aspect of ourselves – which is less openly addressed, but always being impacted. These particular crystals can have a profound effect, by naturally shifting our feelings, relieving stress and boosting temperament.

Here are ten crystals to help improve mood and promote a sense of calm:

- Celestite
- Blue lace agate
- Sunstone
- Citrine
- Clear quartz
- Aquamarine
- Blue topaz
- Obsidian
- Tiger's eye
- Larimar

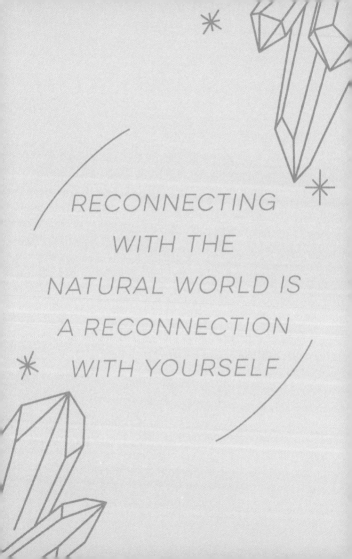

RECONNECTING WITH THE NATURAL WORLD IS A RECONNECTION WITH YOURSELF

# HEALING GEM ELIXIRS

After all this talk of the metaphysical properties of beloved gems, it may come as no surprise that liquids can hold and emit energy as well.

Crystals can impact serums, spritzes and even cleaning products, transforming them into healing elixirs. These crystal solutions can be formulated as sprays to influence the energy of your space. When combined with intention, they can be a useful ritual and further enhance the desired themes of your chosen crystals.

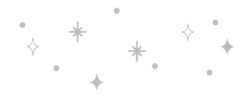

## MAKE YOUR OWN
## CHARGED HOME SPRAY

The optimum time for making your own home spritz is during new and full moons, and the choice will be based on your intentions. Allow a moon-charged crystal, such as rose quartz, to sit for a few hours in spring water, or immerse the crystal in water overnight. If you're soaking the crystal during a full moon, try to keep it within the light of the moon. If you don't wish to soak the crystal, or if the stone you've selected shouldn't be exposed to water, you can simply leave it touching a bowl of water under the moonlight. This water should be exposed to the moon's brightness, to enhance its potency. You could even create a grid with your chosen crystals.

If you have kept a stone submerged, remove the stone and bottle the water in an airtight spray bottle, adding any desired essential oils, such as clary sage, lavender and geranium. Keep this spray on hand for a couple of weeks and spritz regularly, for energetic purification and an intentional uplift in your home.

## PROTECTION WITH CRYSTALS

The energy field that surrounds all living things and emits an energy is sometimes referred to as the "aura." This name is derived from the Greek word, *avra*, meaning "breeze", and is a goddess name in Greek mythology. The aura is a non-visible but emanating energy that some people can feel. You might be able to sense the aura in some circumstances, such as when you're out in nature, but not in others. Crystal wands are known for clearing one's aura, or auric field, particularly wands made from selenite.

Clearing our aura can help us slough off the junk that isn't ours to carry, and it can also help to uplift our aura. As we've witnessed from the historical cataloguing of crystals across cultures, specific stones are used to do this. These shielding stones carry potent energy, especially combined with the intention of their wearer. You'll find them all in the Essential Crystals guide (from page 93), but black tourmaline, shungite and hematite are examples of general stones that offer protective vibrations.

# WRITING WITH CRYSTALS

Writing intentions can be a powerful practice, helping you identify the missing links between where you are and where you're heading. Outside of specific intentions, creating a habit of writing, or a writing ritual, can help formulate the steps towards what you are trying to create.

For example, when you start the process of free writing (writing whatever comes to mind), you might discover you are missing a necessary stage or next step that will draw you closer to your goals or wishes. Or maybe you think you understand how you're feeling about a particular relationship or aspect of your life, but more illumination arises from your writing ritual.

Writing is a terrific practice for gaining clarity and clearing out emotions. Devoting a window of time to pour feelings and thoughts onto the page can help you connect with your heart and inner guidance, and crystals can be easily incorporated into this process.

For each of the writing strategies provided, use the crystals that feel most appropriate for you. Ones that are supportive of your voice (the shade of blue) can be a good place to start. You can incorporate these beauties by carrying, wearing or keeping them in sight throughout your writing exercise. If this turns into a habit of scribbling thoughts, you may even want to designate a particular set of crystals for this.

## WAYS TO WRITE
## WITH CRYSTALS

+ **Stream-of-consciousness writing:** with pen held to paper, start free-form writing. Literally any thought that comes to mind can get jotted down. It doesn't have to make sense, or even be legible. The point is to free yourself from the restraint to be a perfect communicator and tap into what may intuitively rise to the surface. When choosing this method, try incorporating a crystal related to the third eye (see page 36 for a reminder).

◆ **Journaling with prompts:** start your writing with a few questions. You might have some prompts that come to mind, but the following chapter is filled with questions devoted to each of the crystals, so this might be a good place to start. Begin your journaling with the intention to address any underlying concerns and continue forward in healing.

◆ **Journaling towards an intention:** with this, there's no pressure to continually write, as with free-form writing, and there's no real question to answer. Simply write whatever comes to mind and go down the rabbit holes you wish to go down – it's entirely your choice. Based on what you wind up jotting down, notice which themes arise. As you read what you've written, what specific healing is needed? Focus on which crystals you feel will work best with these intentions.

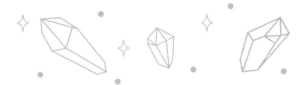

Crystals
amplify the
consciousness.

**SHIRLEY MacLAINE**

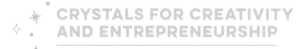

# CRYSTALS FOR CREATIVITY AND ENTREPRENEURSHIP

If you are an entrepreneur, drive, courage and inspiration might come naturally to you. If you are creative, you know the thrill of diving into your artistic pursuits. But whether in business or art, it's likely your inspiration ebbs and flows. During those "down" seasons – when you're feeling lethargic or uninspired – just remember there's a crystal for that.

Citrine or sunstone can put you in an easy-going state to create. If your work needs a heartfelt infusion of passionate energy, trying stones like green calcite or rose quartz might do just the trick. If your work or craft involves public speaking, you may feel inspired by some confidence-boosting stones, like tiger's eye or carnelian. Malachite is also an empowering stone for venturing into uncharted territory in the workplace, or helping you elevate to the position of centre stage.

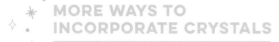

## MORE WAYS TO INCORPORATE CRYSTALS

### OUT IN NATURE

Keeping a healing stone in your hand during a meditative walk is a way to incorporate crystals into your routine. Being in nature while holding a piece of it can produce a soothing effect and help you be present in the moment.

### BREATHWORK

Try holding crystals during a breathwork session. This doesn't need to be too formal a practice – just a few rounds of deep, intentional breathing with your eyes closed will do.

### YOGA

Keeping crystals nearby, or on a corner of your mat, during a yoga practice is another way to add crystals to your active life. Choose stones with meanings that align with your personal objectives, then simply let the stones do what they do.

## CRYSTAL CLASHES

There are some stones that just don't work well together. In some instances, these stones cancel out each other's energies, or simply cause friction. To save yourself a potential headache, let's consider some examples:

### ENERGY VERSUS CALM

In most instances, combining energizing and calming stones will not make sense, for instance, stimulating carnelian with soothing celestite. These are contradicting energies, which support conflicting intentions.

### SLEEP PROBLEMS

Sleeping next to stimulating stones might be counterproductive to your healthy sleep regime. You'll want to try soothing stones instead.

### AMPLIFYING STONES

If you're feeling sensitive to the energy of a certain stone, you might prefer avoiding anything that can amplify it, such as clear quartz. Some stones, such as moldavite, are known to have intense energies, so you may want to avoid combining this with anything if you're just getting acquainted with its energy.

## LACK OF GROUNDING

If you're seeking stability and grounded support, utilizing many upper chakra stones will conflict with your desire for security. Sometimes, at the start of our crystal journey, we surround ourselves with these third eye and crown chakra stones. They're not only beautiful, but they're also easy to find and admire. While beneficial for intuitive support, if you're feeling distracted and have been working with these upper chakra stones, you'll want to seek root chakra stones for balance, to counteract this.

## LACK OF INSIGHT

On the other hand, if you've been feeling stuck in your daily grind and need greater intuitive guidance, you'll want to incorporate more of those high chakra stones, while avoiding grounding stones.

Ultimately, there's no *wrong* way to combine stones, but there are more effective methods to benefit from them.

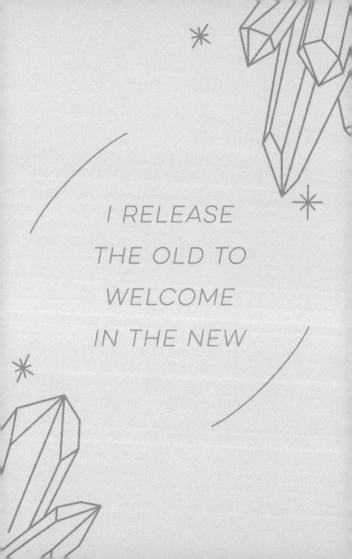

I RELEASE
THE OLD TO
WELCOME
IN THE NEW

## ✦ LOVE AND CRYSTALS

You may have heard the phrase "love spell". This idea of beckoning love towards us is intended to welcome in an energy, as opposed to connecting us to a specific person. If you're seeking connection with a healthy romantic partner, finding sensual compatibility and reciprocity in partnership, a ritual connecting you to the energy of love is another way to utilize crystals.

You will want to find the love stones that speak to you. These might include rose quartz, kunzite, green calcite or peridot – there are many! You can simply incorporate a love crystal into your routine, or accessorize with them. But first, after clearing and cleansing your chosen crystal, set the intention for love without tying it to the necessity of a specific person having to perform this role or function.

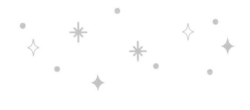

# MONEY STONES

From targeting money mindset blocks to money coaching, rituals around manifesting money are everywhere. In fact, your work routine is a money-making ritual. But there are specific stones that assist in cultivating feelings of abundance, which are recognized for programming with this intention.

Jade, pyrite and peridot are just a few stones you can use for your money intentions. For a practice, start by creating or tweaking your budget, and consider setting an amount you are desiring for a specific project. This will need to be connected with your purpose or something that greatly matters to you, not just a basic desire to have more money. Explore avenues that can support this goal and keep your money stone programmed with your specific intention in a space of work. Depending on the professional skills this requires, you may choose to couple this with stones that support effective communication or self-confidence.

# ✳ SYMBOLISM OF THE HANDS

Just as with colours, cardinal directions and gemstones, there's an energy attached to the left and right sides of ourselves – particularly in the hands. Our left side is connected to themes of receptivity and allowing others to provide, while the right is one of giving and outward action. These two energies intertwined remind us of healthy energy exchange. You can utilize this information for your crystal healing work, particularly in meditation.

When your intention involves being open to receive, try holding your crystals in your left hand, or allow your hand to be open and upright. When your intention is to take action or create something, experiment using your right hand for programming or meditating with your crystals.

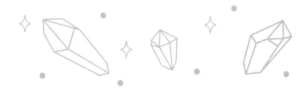

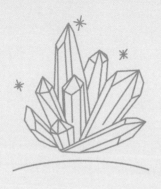

# THERE CAN BE
# DEEP MEANING IN
# SMALL THINGS

# CRYSTALS BY SIGN

In the first century BCE, Jewish historian Josephus believed there was a correlation between the 12 stones in Aaron's breastplate, the 12 months of the year and the 12 signs of the zodiac. Since then, many scholars have acknowledged the crystals that best support the celestial energies of each of the zodiacal signs, including precious and semi-precious stones.

Wearing the stone which corresponds with your star sign is thought to help you embody more of your personal traits and gifts – the things that make you unique. This happens alongside the more specific benefits each of these stones offer. In addition to working with the stones of your own zodiac sign, you could explore the stones and their themes at each time of the year as it unfolds. You may find you tap more naturally into each one's flow of energy during its annual phase, such as aligning with carnelian's drive during the birth of spring, or embracing the protection and support of obsidian for All Hallows' Eve.

## SIGNS OF THE ZODIAC

✦ Aries (March 21 – April 20): bloodstone, carnelian, diamond, ruby.

✦ Taurus (April 21 – May 20): sapphire, golden topaz, rhodonite, emerald.

✦ Gemini (May 21 – June 20): agate, opal, pearl, emerald.

✦ Cancer (June 21 – July 22): ruby, alexandrite, pearl, moonstone.

✦ Leo (July 23 – August 23): peridot, onyx, tiger's eye, amber.

✦ Virgo (August 24 – September 22): sapphire, carnelian, jade, peridot.

✦ Libra (September 23 – October 23): peridot, clear quartz, opal, lapis lazuli.

✦ Scorpio (October 24 – November 22): topaz, citrine, aquamarine, obsidian.

✦ Sagittarius (November 23 – December 20): turquoise, topaz, citrine, tanzanite.

✦ Capricorn (December 21 – January 19): garnet, ruby, sapphire, blue topaz.

✦ Aquarius (January 20 – February 18): amethyst, garnet, labradorite.

✦ Pisces (February 19 – March 20): turquoise, fluorite, amethyst, aquamarine.

*Nature is the*
*purest portal*
*to inner peace.*

ANGIE WEILAND-CROSBY

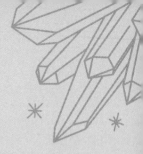

# CHAPTER FOUR:

## ESSENTIAL CRYSTALS

From A–Z, the following pages will serve as a jumping-off point for your crystal exploration journey. While more than 4,000 different crystals have been discovered and classified, here are some of the most popular. For each, you'll learn about a practice, as well as their unique origins, individual themes and ways to work with their energy. You'll also discover the chakra associations for your healing rituals.

Notice which crystal names attract you, prior to reading their attributes. You might be intrigued to explore further – even before the healing magic of the stones reaches your hand...

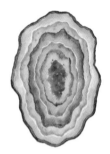

# AGATE

CHAKRA: **Root, heart, third eye, crown**

ORIGIN: **Sicily**

THEMES: **Clarity and grounding**

Agate supports mental clarity, calmness and ease. It helps stabilize the root chakra and comes in a variety of different hues, including moss agate and blue lace agate, along with shades of brown and purple, with the colour suggesting the chakra it targets.

## HEALING TIPS

REFLECTION: In which area of life do you need greater clarity?

AFFIRMATION: I trust my intuition and make decisions with ease.

PRACTICE: With the energy of clarity and grounding, agate is a wonderful stone to keep in the workplace in the form of a slab, loose stones or decorative art. Wherever you need the most mental focus for decision making, keep agate close for support and stability.

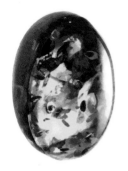

# AMBER

CHAKRA: **Sacral and solar plexus**

ORIGIN: **Germany, Poland, Russia, UK**

THEMES: **Purification and protection**

This rich gold stone often looks like crystallized honey, because it is fossilized resin from pine trees. Just as resin protects the trees, amber is also used for protection. This stone is attributed with uplifting mood, reducing inflammation and ushering in positive experiences.

## HEALING TIPS

REFLECTION: Where do you feel tightness or inflammation in your body?

AFFIRMATION: I welcome in peace and relaxation.

PRACTICE: Perform a healing meditation using amber. Starting with a few cleansing breaths, sip a soothing herbal tea, such as chamomile, and indulge in a salt bath, using natural lavender oil, all with amber by your side.

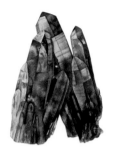

# AMETHYST

CHAKRA: **Third eye and crown**

ORIGIN: **Brazil, Greece, India, Russia, Uruguay, USA, Zambia**

THEMES: **Enlightenment and protection**

A memorable purple stone, amethyst is tied to spiritual protection. It supports the gaining of clarity and, historically, symbolized luxury and abundance. When you're carrying the weight of the world, this is terrific for renewed perspective and cleansing energy.

## HEALING TIPS

REFLECTION: What can be eliminated in my routine to support my healing?

AFFIRMATION: I am open to receiving divine guidance for my highest good.

PRACTICE: If you don't have a routine meditation practice, start with ten minutes, preferably in the morning, for seven consecutive days. Keep amethyst close by and set the intention for protection and divine connection. Consider keeping a journal, writing anything that arises.

# AQUAMARINE

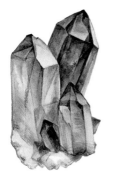

CHAKRA: **Third eye and crown**

ORIGIN: **Afghanistan, Brazil, India, Ireland, Mexico, Pakistan, Russia, USA, Zimbabwe**

THEMES: **Clarity and divinity**

Ranging from clear to opaque, this sea-evoking crystal brings an immediate sense of calm. Known for reducing stress and relaxing the mind, aquamarine is a wonderful companion for meditation. Historically, it was carried by sailors to protect them from drowning.

## HEALING TIPS

REFLECTION: What recent topic or event has left my mind racing?

AFFIRMATION: I am deserving of peace and freedom.

PRACTICE: Choose a time of day when you can devote five to ten minutes for peace and relaxation, without any obligations or interruptions. If you need an alert or reminder, put it on your calendar. Let aquamarine be your signal for serenity.

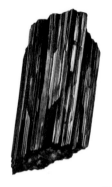

# BLACK TOURMALINE

CHAKRA: **Root**

ORIGIN: **Brazil, Germany, Madagascar, Mozambique, Namibia, Nigeria, Sri Lanka, USA, Zambia**

THEMES: **Shielding and purifying**

All forms of tourmaline, including black tourmaline, are powerful transmuters of energy. Despite its connection with the root, this cleanses all chakras. It's great for warding off bad vibes and assisting with uplifting energy.

## HEALING TIPS

REFLECTION: Are you clinging to emotional residue from your past?

AFFIRMATION: I am supported in the transmuting of energy that doesn't align with my highest good.

PRACTICE: Hold black tourmaline while consciously releasing stuck energy and hurt feelings. Throughout this process, surrender to whatever floats into your awareness. Follow up with an uplifting practice, thought or intention. Clear your space before and after your practice.

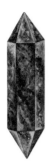

# BLOODSTONE

CHAKRA: **Root**

ORIGIN: **Australia, Brazil, China, Czech Republic, India, Russia**

THEMES: **Courage and alignment**

Bloodstone is a dynamic stone, encouraging stability in times of change and healing. Its protective attributes support the navigation of tricky environments – this is so we can discover the relationships that are most beneficial. Bloodstone supports well-being, stamina and the courage to take a fresh, nurturing path.

## HEALING TIPS

REFLECTION: What's keeping you feeling stuck or small?

AFFIRMATION: I am worthy of feeling supported in my connections and courageous on my path.

PRACTICE: Practice yoga, dance, jiu-jitsu, or anything that requires you to find presence in your body. Keep bloodstone as a reminder of this sensation and to illuminate your inner warrior!

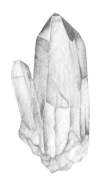

# BLUE TOPAZ

CHAKRA: **Throat**

ORIGIN: **Australia, India,
Mexico, Pakistan,
South Africa, Sri Lanka, USA**

THEMES: **Calm
and visualization**

When we need a spark of clarity, this soft blue gem helps us find it. Blue topaz supports the softer side of life and is healing for the nervous system. It also assists with improving communication.

## HEALING TIPS

REFLECTION: In which connection do I need to seek clarity?

AFFIRMATION: I communicate my desires with ease.

PRACTICE: On a new moon, create a vision board or write out intentions. Create a vision that aligns with feelings of satisfaction and fulfilment. Throughout this process, keep blue topaz with you. Place the stone where you are actively creating this future vision, as a reminder and to support your process.

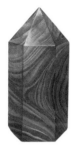

# CARNELIAN

CHAKRA: **Sacral**

ORIGIN: **Brazil, Egypt, Germany, India, Indonesia, Iraq, Russia, Uruguay, USA**

THEMES: **Passion and inspiration**

When we're feeling lethargic, carnelian boosts vitality and helps cultivate creativity. Its vivid colour ranges from bright orange to deep red. Look to carnelian for support in materializing aspirations and connecting with your inner drive.

## HEALING TIPS

REFLECTION: What single action can I take today to contribute to my success?

AFFIRMATION: I move towards my goals with courage and excitement.

PRACTICE: On the next new moon, write your intentions around a new goal or creative project. Write the first steps you need to take. As you move forwards with this new project, keep carnelian in the form of a loose stone or bracelet with you.

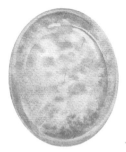

# CELESTITE

CHAKRA: **Throat**

ORIGIN: **Egypt, Libya, Madagascar, Mexico, Peru, Poland, UK**

THEMES: **Truth and intuition**

Celestite – a serene, pale blue – supports conflict resolution and inner peace. Tied to dreams, it assists in connecting with the angelic realm and cultivating deep clarity. As it helps clear intuitive blockages, celestite dissolves obstacles in communication and facilitates mutual understanding.

## HEALING TIPS

REFLECTION: What can I do to achieve greater peace in my relationships?

AFFIRMATION: I find peace, harmony and vulnerability in my relationships.

PRACTICE: Keep celestite on your bedside table and start a dream journal. Practice one specific action to support your bedtime ritual, such as avoiding afternoon caffeine or reducing nightly screen time.

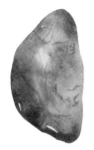

# CHAROITE

CHAKRA: **Crown**

ORIGIN: **Russia**

THEMES: **Transformation and clarity**

A rare purple stone, this is potent and assists in seasons of transition. Tied to the crown chakra, it's known for helping us find connection to our higher selves. If you're experiencing a mindset block, or need to see things from an elevated perspective, use charoite to eliminate blockages in the crown, enabling you to see differently.

## HEALING TIPS

REFLECTION: When it comes to my responsibilities, where do I need to lighten the load?

AFFIRMATION: I can open myself to potential breakthroughs and divine guidance.

PRACTICE: In a meditative state, place charoite over your third eye. Before this process, set an intention for divine guidance for your highest good.

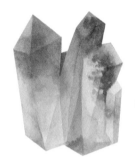

# CITRINE

CHAKRA: **Solar plexus**

ORIGIN: **Africa, France, Greece, Madagascar, Russia, Scotland, Spain, USA**

THEMES: **Joy and empowerment**

This champagne-hued crystal is a builder of healthy confidence. When you've seen yourself through a faulty lens, this is a powerful healing stone. Look to citrine for elevating joy, eliminating negativity and redirecting your focus.

## HEALING TIPS

REFLECTION: Where have I been over-investing my energy?

AFFIRMATION: I am worthy of moving in the direction of my dreams.

PRACTICE: Keep citrine on your desk, next to your bed, or somewhere close at hand when you need a boost of uplifting energy. Allow this sunny gem to remind you to seek joy in the present moment and tap into your inner radiance.

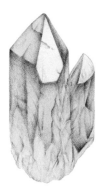

# CLEAR QUARTZ

CHAKRA: **All**

ORIGIN: **Brazil, China, India, Japan, USA**

THEMES: **Balance and amplification**

Clear quartz is a powerhouse crystal with a range of uses, including amplifying the energy of other crystals. It is often used in crystal grids, and it absorbs negative energies in a space while amplifying positive vibes.

## HEALING TIPS

REFLECTION: In which space do I need to infuse more positivity?

AFFIRMATION: I move with intentionality and benefit from clear focus on my passions.

PRACTICE: In preparation for an intuitive exercise, pick up a few different clear quartz stones. After cleaning and clearing your home, walk through and place these where you intuitively feel guided to leave them.

# JADE

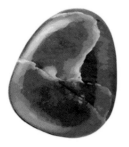

CHAKRA: **Heart**

ORIGIN: **Canada, China, Guyana, Myanmar, New Zealand, Russia, USA**

THEMES: **Spirituality and abundance**

Confucius ascribed jade with the qualities of virtue, wisdom and truth. Prized in indigenous American and Chinese cultures, it has also been associated with nature, growth, fertility, love and money.

## HEALING TIPS

REFLECTION: Where are you being dishonest with yourself about the value you have to offer?

AFFIRMATION: I am worthy.

PRACTICE: Keep a close eye on your budget over the course of a month. Wear jade daily and do affirmation work around your value. Be open to realizing where you might be undervaluing yourself.

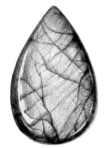

# LABRADORITE

CHAKRA: **Third eye**

ORIGIN: **Canada, Finland, Greenland, Italy, Russia, Scandinavia**

THEMES: **Intuition and clarity**

This mystical blue stone has an iridescent quality that shifts colour with movement. Labradorite supports third eye vision and revelation. When you're feeling disconnected from your intuitive nature, labradorite is a perfect go-to crystal for reconnection and lucidity.

## HEALING TIPS

REFLECTION: Which thought pattern or obsession is clouding your judgement – and what needs releasing to see anew?

AFFIRMATION: I release my present perception and accept heightened awareness of the truth.

PRACTICE: Allow yourself time and space in a tranquil environment. Meditate with labradorite placed on your third eye. Keep a journal nearby in case something fresh comes to light.

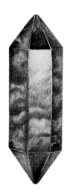

# LAPIS LAZULI

CHAKRA: **Third eye**

ORIGIN: **Afghanistan, Chile, Egypt, Italy, Middle East, Russia**

THEMES: **Empowerment and protection**

An electric and empowering blue stone, this helps us heal trauma, grief and throat chakra blockages. Also affiliated with the third eye, lapis lazuli is known for intuitive properties that provide protection for its wearers. It supports a regal, confident pep in your step!

## HEALING TIPS

REFLECTION: What would I do if I had no perceived obstacles on my path?

AFFIRMATION: With courage, I express my authentic truth.

PRACTICE: If you're in need of a little confidence, wear lapis lazuli. Begin a daily morning meditation practice and connect with the themes of lapis lazuli in your conscious link to the divine.

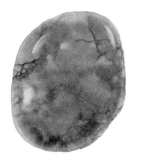

# LARIMAR

CHAKRA: **Throat**

ORIGIN: **Dominican Republic**

THEMES: **Serenity and purification**

A rare crystal, larimar carries a strong feminine energy. With cool ocean tones suggesting a reassuring calm, it helps to quell anxiety and bridge the gap between our true desires and the expression of them in our own voice.

## HEALING TIPS

REFLECTION: Where in my body do I feel tension or anxiety?

AFFIRMATION: I am free and calm in my body and mind.

PRACTICE: Spend a couple of weeks noticing the physical sensations in your body in certain environments. Keep larimar with you throughout this time, setting the intention to release stuck energy and connect with your truth.

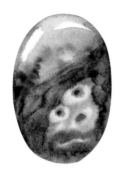

# MALACHITE

CHAKRA: **Heart**

ORIGIN: **Democratic Republic of Congo, Romania, Russia, Zambia**

THEMES: **Transformation and self-assurance**

Malachite's rich, vibrant green mirrors its theme of empowerment. In addition to heart connectivity, it's a stone of protection and transformation. When you feel weak-willed or insecure and you need to connect with yourself, receive the support of malachite.

## HEALING TIPS

REFLECTION: What's one step I can take towards my vision?

AFFIRMATION: Unapologetically, I move towards my heart's desire.

PRACTICE: During a new moon, identify a project you've struggled to get off the ground. Identify how you envision the project in its completed state. Use malachite to establish your short-term plan to support your long-term intention.

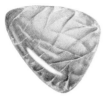

# MOONSTONE

Moonstone is tied to intuition, dreams and the moon. This milky-hued stone comes in cream, white, blue and green tones and is an excellent go-to crystal for clarity.

## HEALING TIPS

REFLECTION: Are the opinions of others drowning out your intuitive clarity?

AFFIRMATION: I have faith in my intuition to guide me, and I turn within for answers.

PRACTICE: If you're in the habit of checking with others before listening to your inner wisdom, try a regular writing routine, meditation practice, prayer, or another way to connect with your intuition before seeking the opinions of other people.

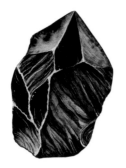

# OBSIDIAN

ORIGIN: **Argentina, Canada, Chile, Greece, Guatemala, Hungary, Iceland, Italy, Japan, Kenya, Mexico, New Zealand, Russia, USA**

THEMES: **Protection and authenticity**

This slick, opaque black stone is terrific for boundary work. When you're working to disconnect from over-caring about the opinions of others, keep obsidian close. It's one of the more powerful protection stones, sometimes used in gardens to safeguard a home.

## HEALING TIPS

REFLECTION: Where do you need to assert better boundaries through communication and removing yourself from situations?

AFFIRMATION: I am safe and secure being true to myself.

PRACTICE: With a piece of obsidian on a necklace or bracelet, set the intention for peaceful, loving connections to surround you. Wear this consistently.

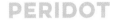

# PERIDOT

CHAKRA: **Heart**

ORIGIN: **Australia, Brazil, China, Egypt, Kenya, Mexico, Myanmar, Norway, Pakistan, USA**

THEMES: **Prosperity and happiness**

Peridot was a beloved favourite of Queen Cleopatra, who wore it for its beauty and powers of protection. With a lush shade of green, peridot evokes feelings of rebirth, springtime, joy and abundance, imbuing wearers with confidence and joy.

## HEALING TIPS

REFLECTION: What part of your life is hungry for rebirth?

AFFIRMATION: Through heart-aligned living, I welcome prosperity, joy and protection into my life.

PRACTICE: Place peridot over the heart in a heart-chakra focused meditation. Then, wear it as an amulet or ring to remind you of healing and prosperity as you venture forth on your path to abundance.

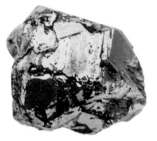

# PYRITE

CHAKRA: **Solar plexus**

ORIGIN: **Italy, Kazakhstan, Peru, Spain, USA**

THEMES: **Prosperity and vitality**

This gold metallic cube radiates the energy of abundance. When you have budget and money goals in mind, this is a stone to keep with you. It's also great for infusing creative spark into daily tasks and reconnecting with your willpower.

## HEALING TIPS

REFLECTION: What money stories are standing between me and my perception of my value?

AFFIRMATION: I am abundant and empowered.

PRACTICE: Keep pyrite in plain sight within your workspace – next to a computer or where you need that extra boost to keep going when you feel your energy levels dip. Allow its presence to increase your vitality.

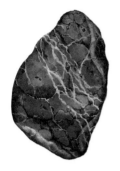

# RED JASPER

CHAKRA: **Root**

ORIGIN: **Brazil, France, Germany, India, Russia, USA**

THEMES: **Presence and stability**

This red clay-coloured stone reinforces root chakra themes of security and pragmatism. On our healing journeys we can be distracted by anxious thoughts, but red jasper brings tranquillity and present-moment awareness. This back-to-earth pull helps us step off the psychological hamster wheel.

## HEALING TIPS

REFLECTION: What's one step I can take towards greater physical or financial stability?

AFFIRMATION: I find calmness and presence in this moment.

PRACTICE: When you're feeling angsty or having trouble concentrating, wear red jasper. Walk barefoot on the grass. Breathe. Notice all the sensations in your body, here and now.

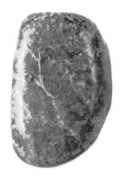

# RHODONITE

CHAKRA: **Heart**

ORIGIN: **Australia, Canada, Finland, Japan, Madagascar, Mexico, Russia, South Africa, Sweden, Tanzania, USA**

THEMES: **Forgiveness and restoration**

Known as the "rescue stone", this powerful pink crystal is intended for mending wounds of the heart. A go-to when release feels particularly tough, it's also one of the top stones for emotional healing and supporting healthy relationships.

## HEALING TIPS

REFLECTION: How can I reframe forgiveness as acceptance?

AFFIRMATION: I reclaim my power.

PRACTICE: To work with this stone's sensual and romantic energies, place it in your bedroom for the intention of relationship restoration.

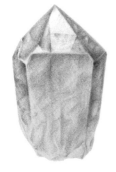

# ROSE QUARTZ

CHAKRA: **Heart**

ORIGIN: **Brazil, India, Japan, Madagascar, South Africa, USA**

THEMES: **Self-love and compassion**

This popular, blush-coloured stone's most prevalent theme is self-love and it's connected to our receptivity of love. It helps with eradicating pain and clearing blockages, and can assist with healing trauma and grief, as well as dissipating feelings of resentment or jealousy.

## HEALING TIPS

REFLECTION: In what ways do I show compassion to myself?

AFFIRMATION: I am open to receiving love.

PRACTICE: The subtle energy of rose quartz makes it a wonderful stone to wear. While doing so, focus on your willingness to receive love instead of performing for it. Couple this with a healing affirmation every day.

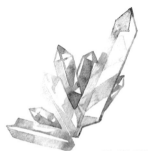

# SELENITE

CHAKRA: **Third eye and crown**

ORIGIN: **Mexico, Australia, Greece, Madagascar, USA**

THEMES: **Uplift and purification**

In appearance and energy, translucent selenite has an angelic quality. It helps clear the energies of other crystals and our auric field, working in a similar way to clearing herbs. When used in meditation, it can provide insights and greater levels of self-awareness.

## HEALING TIPS

REFLECTION: Am I carrying weight that is not mine to carry?

AFFIRMATION: I release all energies that are not mine to hold.

PRACTICE: Keep a selenite wand handy for clearing energy. After challenging moments and conversations, expel the emotions in a healthy way — such as speaking or writing your truth. Then, clear the energy with your selenite wand.

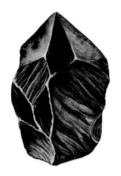

# SHUNGITE

CHAKRA: **Root**

ORIGIN: **Russia**

THEMES: **Shielding and purifying**

This opaque black stone is a powerful protector which is physically and energetically detoxifying. It guards against electromagnetic frequencies and harmful digital vibes. It's a strong grounding stone that helps release negativity, opening the door for more uplifting, positive energy.

## HEALING TIPS

REFLECTION: When it comes to time spent on devices, could you benefit from being more selective?

AFFIRMATION: I am guarded against negativity and bad vibes.

PRACTICE: With strong technological clearing capacity, keep shungite near your electronics. You might consider resting your phone on a shungite cube or storing it near your laptop.

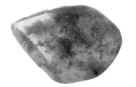

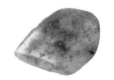

# SUNSTONE

CHAKRA: **Sacral**

ORIGIN: **Canada, China, Congo, India, Mexico, Norway, Sri Lanka, Tanzania, USA**

THEMES: **Creativity and happiness**

A sunny shade of orange or red, sunstone is an invigorating stone that inspires strong self-love and vivacity. This can be used for reigniting your passion in artistic endeavours. To amplify positivity, surround yourself with the joy-filled vibrations of sunstone!

## HEALING TIPS

REFLECTION: How can I intentionally plan for more joy this week?

AFFIRMATION: I actively invite more joy into my life.

PRACTICE: What did you enjoy doing as a child? Gather a group of friends for a games night, plan a picnic or pick up a guitar, even if it's been ages since you did so. Whichever activity you desire, use sunstone to invite more play into your life.

# TIGER'S EYE

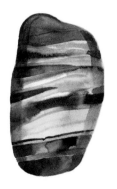

CHAKRA: **Root, sacral and solar plexus**

ORIGIN: **Australia, Brazil, China, India, Myanmar, Nambia, South Africa, USA**

THEMES: **Courage and protection**

This toasty-brown stone has a silky lustre and is grounded, while stimulating. It's a powerful stone of transmutation, helping transform self-doubt into self-assurance. When you're seeking forward momentum, be ready for the change facilitated by tiger's eye.

## HEALING TIPS

REFLECTION: Which past experience needs acceptance for me to reclaim my strength and move forwards in a positive way?

AFFIRMATION: I release the old and step into the new for my highest good.

PRACTICE: Tiger's eye is an excellent stone to wear for a combination of shielding unwanted vibes and stimulating creative energies.

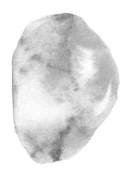

# TURQUOISE

CHAKRA: **Throat**

ORIGIN: **Afghanistan, Australia, Chile, China, Egypt, Iran, Mexico, USA**

THEMES: **Truth and ease**

Like its vibrant blue suggests, turquoise is a calming stone. Wearing turquoise is thought to offer soothing balm from external influences and facilitate the emergence of essential truths. It is connected to our intuitive understanding and carries an ability to guide us out of undesirable situations through honest communication.

## HEALING TIPS

REFLECTION: Where are am I silencing my voice for fear of being judged?

AFFIRMATION: My truth is always worthy of being expressed.

PRACTICE: In a meditative resting position, place turquoise over the throat chakra. Following your meditation, complete a journaling exercise around themes that may have arisen.

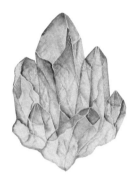

# YELLOW TOPAZ

CHAKRA: **Solar plexus**

ORIGIN: **Brazil, Mexico, Russia, USA**

THEMES: **Stimulation and inspiration**

Vibrant yellow topaz brings radiant energy to our creative endeavours. Its happy-go-lucky vibes are subtle and encourage action towards our vision, manifesting new beginnings and elevating energy from low or depressed to pleasure and delight.

## HEALING TIPS

REFLECTION: Which endeavours are draining my energy?

AFFIRMATION: I prioritize my joy and creativity.

PRACTICE: Sitting with yellow topaz, explore topics of creativity. When you were a child, what did you love to do? When was the last time you explored that activity? How can you prioritize play? Explore these themes to bring more inspiration and fun into your routine.

# CONCLUSION

Since dipping your toes into the world of crystals, how has your understanding of gemstones changed? Now you have an awareness of how to use them, beyond displaying or wearing them as pretty trinkets, will you begin to incorporate them into your daily life?

Through practice, you'll develop your own relationship with these beautiful pieces of history, discovering new crystals beyond those we've covered here. Your newfound crystal knowledge is powerful – their collective history can encourage reverence for those who came before and appreciation for nature's bounty, but your own intuition is your ultimate guide.

Even with an arsenal of crystal knowledge, your greatest asset in performing personal healing work is developing a more intimate relationship with yourself. Your inner wisdom is a resource for your growth, healing and expansion – use it and enjoy the journey!

# CRYSTALS INDEX

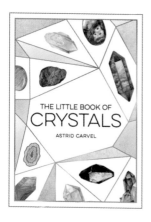

## THE LITTLE BOOK OF CRYSTALS

A Beginner's Guide to Crystal Healing

Astrid Carvel

Paperback

ISBN: 978-1-78685-959-4

Learn how to select and maintain your crystals as well as basic techniques for crystal meditation, balancing chakras and simple ways to bring harmony to mind, body and spirit with these natural treasures. Discover over 50 crystals, their unique properties and how to make use of their power in everyday life. There is a crystal for every occasion.

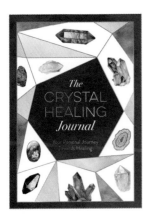

THE CRYSTAL HEALING JOURNAL

Track Your Personal Journey Towards Healing
with Crystals

Astrid Carvel

Paperback

ISBN: 978-1-80007-677-8

A beautifully designed guided journal, with thoughtful
prompts to guide you through different crystal-healing
practices using 30 essential restorative stones, and to
track and your journey towards better health and well-
being. Includes a history of crystals and tips on how to
choose, cleanse, charge and care for your collection.

Have you enjoyed this book?
If so, find us on
Facebook at **Summersdale Publishers**,
on Twitter at **@Summersdale** and on
Instagram and TikTok at **@summersdalebooks**
and get in touch.
We'd love to hear from you!

## www.summersdale.com